ITRAVIL

Unlocking the secrets of successful
weight loss

DR. DAVID OXFORD

form or by any means, including photocopying, recording or other electronic or mechanical methods, without the prior written permission of the publisher, except in the case of brief quotations embodied in critical reviews and certain other noncommercial uses permitted by copyright law.
Copyright © 2024 DR. David oxford

TABLE OF CONTENTS

INTRODUCTION

Itravil is a pharmaceutical company that operates in the field of weight control, namely in the nexus of pharmacology and health. Created primarily to support people on their weight-loss journey, Itravil is a combination of medical knowledge and scientific research. Itravil is essentially a drug that is part of a certain class of medications called anorexigenics, which are designed to control hunger and aid in efforts to achieve a healthier body weight.

In the current health and wellness scene, where obesity and associated health issues are widespread, Itravil appears as a pharmacological option that provides a more sophisticated approach to managing weight. Its formulation, which aims to address the intricate interplay between physiological elements controlling body weight, is based on knowledge of neurochemistry and metabolic processes.

Itravil is a possible ally for those starting weight loss programs since it interferes with the regulation of neurotransmitters and signaling pathways that control hunger and fullness. This intervention is designed to encourage a long-term decrease in calorie intake, which will facilitate a slow and steady advancement toward weight-related objectives.

Itravil's development is rooted in a dedication to evidence-based medicine, which is supported by thorough research and clinical trials. The addition of this drug to the therapeutic repertoire demonstrates a commitment to developing treatment approaches for those dealing with the difficulties associated with being overweight.

In addition to its pharmaceutical component, Itravil emphasizes the significance of a comprehensive strategy for managing weight. Its entry into the healthcare continuum promotes a multimodal approach that includes lifestyle changes, dietary advice, frequent physical activity, and medication intervention.

The pharmacological characteristics of Itravil, as well as its uses, dosage, administration, adverse reactions, drug interactions, precautions, and other relevant information, will all be thoroughly explored in the parts that follow in this publication. The goal of this thorough review is to provide patients and medical professionals with the knowledge they need to make well-informed decisions about using Itravil as part of their weight-management program.

All things considered, the arrival of Itravil on the therapeutic scene is a positive development in the continuous quest for better health, offering a useful instrument to those who are dedicated to their quest for reduced body weight and enhanced health.

PHARMACOLOGICAL PROPERTIES

As a pharmaceutical agent, it predominantly affects the central nervous system by way of a complex interaction with neurotransmitters and neurochemical pathways. Clobenzorex hydrochloride is the active component of Itravil, and the drug's pharmacological characteristics help it play a part in weight management.

As a prodrug, sympathomimetic amine clobenzorex is transformed by the body's metabolism into amphetamine, which is its active form. Hepatic enzymes aid in this conversion, which results in the release of amphetamine, a stimulant of the central nervous system. Numerous pharmacological effects follow, including the regulation of neurotransmitters including serotonin, dopamine, and norepinephrine.

Itravil functions primarily as an appetite suppressant with central action. It lessens the feeling of hunger by stimulating the hypothalamic satiety area and increasing norepinephrine release. By influencing the eating habits of those undergoing weight management, this method of action seeks to reduce caloric intake.

Moreover, some people using Itravil report an overall improvement in mood, which may be attributed to the modulation of dopamine levels. A neurotransmitter linked to reward and pleasure, dopamine is involved in mood regulation. Itravil's effect on dopamine levels may give people more psychological support as they deal with the difficulties of changing their lifestyles and losing weight.

Itravil's pharmacological profile goes beyond how it interacts with neurotransmitters. Moreover, it causes sympathomimetic reactions, which raise blood pressure and heart rate. When determining if Itravil is appropriate for a given patient, particularly one who already has a cardiovascular disease, healthcare practitioners should take these cardiovascular consequences into account.

Itravil may also have an effect on thermogenesis, which would encourage a greater energy expenditure. By addressing both sides of the energy balance equation—reducing calorie intake through appetite suppression and increasing calorie expenditure through increased metabolic activity—this feature contributes to its overall role in helping weight loss attempts.

Knowing Itravil's pharmacokinetics is essential, just like with other pharmaceutical intervention. Following oral treatment, clobenzorex is rapidly absorbed; peak plasma concentrations are obtained in a few of hours. The medication is metabolized by the liver, and the majority of its metabolites are eliminated through urine.

Itravil's pharmacological characteristics highlight its comprehensive strategy for managing weight. Itravil promises to help people lose weight and keep it off by modifying neurotransmitters, appetite suppression, and sympathetic responses. It works as a pharmaceutical supplement to complete lifestyle improvements. The complex interactions between these pharmacological systems provide the foundation for comprehending the drug's possible effects on people who are trying to lose weight.

INDICATIONS AND USAGE

The drug Itravil, which is at the forefront of weight management treatments, has many indications that are centered around tackling the intricate and multidimensional problems related to obesity. Itravil is a pharmacological instrument that should only be used under certain conditions when its special profile fits the treatment objectives of those trying to reach and keep a healthier body weight. This in-depth investigation will focus on the subtle signs and proper use of Itravil in relation to weight control.

Signs and symptoms:

Itravil is primarily indicated for the management of obesity. A major global health concern is obesity, a chronic medical condition marked by an excessive buildup of body fat. Obesity patients frequently have a higher chance of getting comorbid conditions such as type 2 diabetes, cardiovascular disease, and musculoskeletal problems. In this case, the function of Itravil is to act as an adjuvant therapy, helping people lose extra weight when non-pharmacological methods have not worked well enough on their own. It is important to remember that Itravil is meant to be used in conjunction with a comprehensive weight management plan, not as a stand-alone treatment. Itravil's indications cover situations in which dietary adjustments and increased physical activity, for example, have not produced the desired weight loss or have proven difficult to maintain.

Guidelines for Usage:

It is essential to perform a comprehensive evaluation of the patient's medical history, risk factors, and general health before starting Itravil therapy. Cardiovascular health should also be evaluated because Itravil's sympathomimetic effects may affect blood pressure and heart rate. When prescribing Itravil, a doctor should carefully weigh the advantages and disadvantages of the medication while also taking the patient's unique needs and circumstances into account.
The degree of obesity, the patient's response to past weight-management techniques, and any underlying medical issues are all taken into account when determining the recommended dosage of Itravil.

Usually, a cautious starting dosage is used to enable close observation of the patient's response and tolerance.

Itravil is usually taken orally, and because of its quick absorption, it takes effect somewhat quickly. To reduce potential adverse effects and maximize appetite suppression, healthcare experts may suggest breaking up the daily dosage into smaller amounts to be taken throughout the day.

It is imperative that healthcare providers inform patients about the significance of following recommended dosages and the possible repercussions of noncompliance as part of the usage instructions. Patients should also be made aware of the anticipated length of their treatment as well as the necessity of routine follow-up visits to assess progress, resolve any issues, and modify the treatment plan as needed.

Patient Selection and Related Factors:

The choice to recommend Itravil requires a careful assessment of the patient's appropriateness. Those who qualify for Itravil should have a body mass index (BMI) that is higher than a specific threshold, which usually denotes moderate to severe obesity.

Additionally, those who were given the option to get Itravil therapy had to show that they were committed to changing their diets and increasing their physical activity.

Patients who already have cardiovascular disease should be given extra caution because Itravil's sympathomimetic effects may increase their risks. Under these circumstances, the decision-making process should be guided by a comprehensive risk-benefit analysis, and close monitoring of cardiovascular markers is crucial during the course of treatment.

Given that there is insufficient evidence to conclude that Itravil is safe to use during pregnancy, women who are or may become pregnant should be advised of the significance of using contraception while undergoing treatment. Healthcare professionals should also be on the lookout for any possible drug interactions, particularly with prescriptions that could alter serotonin or blood pressure.

Observation and Adverse Event Handling:

Ensuring the safety and efficacy of Itravil medication requires frequent patient monitoring. This involves routine evaluations of cardiovascular markers, the rate of weight loss, and any possible negative effects. Healthcare professionals should continue to be on the lookout for symptoms of raised blood pressure, fast heart rate, and mood swings.

Timely modifications to the treatment plan may be required in the event of adverse events or inadequate response. This can entail adjusting the dosage, stopping abruptly, or looking into different weight-management techniques. In order to promote proactive care and reduce potential problems, patient education about the identification and reporting of adverse events is essential.

Current weight-management techniques are deeply entwined with the indications and use of Itravil. Itravil is marketed as an additional treatment for people struggling with obesity, providing a pharmaceutical option to support lifestyle changes. Prescription of Itravil requires careful evaluation of patient suitability, weighing of advantages and disadvantages, and continuous monitoring to guarantee safety and effectiveness.

Itravil is proof of how pharmaceutical developments can be included into holistic health practices, even as the field of managing obesity management changes. Through its distinct pharmacological characteristics, Itravil tackles the intricacies of obesity, making it an invaluable instrument for medical practitioners collaborating with individuals dedicated to achieving weight loss and enhanced health.

DOSAGE AND ADMINISTRATION

A sophisticated grasp of Itravil's dosage and administration guidelines is essential for its wise and efficient use. Itravil is a drug intended to help with weight management, therefore determining the right dosage is essential to maximizing therapeutic benefits and lowering dangers. This thorough investigation will cover the specifics of Itravil's dosage, the variables that affect dosage calculation, and the recommendations for its administration.

Considering Dosage:

Itravil dose determination is a sensitive procedure that requires a customized method that considers the patient's response to the medication, the degree of obesity, and individual features. During this decision-making process, healthcare providers are crucial because they use their clinical knowledge to balance the best possible treatment outcomes with the least amount of side effects.

When using Itravil orally, the recommended initial dosage usually varies between 16 and 37.5 mg per day. Healthcare providers, however, might start patients on a lesser dosage of medication, particularly if they have a higher susceptibility to sympathomimetic drugs or are more likely to experience cardiovascular problems.

The patient's response and tolerance serve as guidelines for subsequent dosage modifications. Titration may entail little dosage increases to enable a steady adaptation to the effects of the medicine. Dosage modifications must be made carefully, taking into account the patient's overall health, the rate of weight reduction, and the existence of any side effects.

Customized Method:

Individualization is more than just choosing a dosage initially. The key to using Itravil therapy effectively is still customizing it to each patient's specific needs and characteristics. This personalized approach is influenced by the patient's age, co-occurring conditions, concurrent drugs, and lifestyle choices.

For example, elderly individuals may need more cautious dosing because of possible age-related changes in medication metabolism and heightened vulnerability to specific side effects. On the other hand, younger people might be able to handle bigger dosages, although caution is needed to prevent overstimulating the central nervous system.

Individuals with several medical disorders, particularly those related to the heart, require a careful evaluation of the risks and benefits. Itravil's sympathomimetic effects may affect blood pressure and heart rate, necessitating close observation and possibly affecting dosage choices in some situations.

Dosage Forms and Procedures:

Oral dosage forms, such as pills or capsules, are the usual forms in which Itravil is supplied. The patient's preference, the simplicity of administration, and the accessibility of particular formulations are some of the variables that may influence the dosage form selection. The timing of administration of tablets or capsules may vary depending on the patient's lifestyle and unique response to the prescription. Typically, these forms of administration are taken with water.

It is advised to take Itravil prior to meals in order to maximize its ability to decrease hunger. This deliberate scheduling corresponds with the drug's mode of action, which reduces appetite and allows for a decrease in caloric intake. To reduce possible adverse effects and maximize hunger control, the daily dosage may also be divided into smaller increments and taken throughout the day.

Treatment Duration:

Since Itravil is not meant to be used continuously, the length of treatment should be carefully addressed. It is usually advised to utilize medication for a short period of time in order to prevent tolerance and possible reliance. Depending on how well a patient is following their lifestyle changes and how quickly they are losing weight, medical professionals may prescribe Itravil for a few weeks or months.

The patient and the healthcare professional consult together to decide whether to stop taking Itravil. To reduce the consequences of withdrawal and make the switch to alternate weight-management techniques easier, the dosage may be gradually tapered.

Patient Instruction:

Achieving treatment success requires educating patients on the right dosage and way to administer Itravil. Patient education should include a thorough comprehension of the recommended dosage, the significance of following the recommended schedule, and any possible side effects that call for immediate contact with medical professionals.

Patients need to understand the need of making lifestyle adjustments, such as eating better and exercising more, as essential parts of their weight-loss journey. Patients and healthcare providers feel more like a team when there is open communication regarding the treatment plan's collaborative character, realistic weight loss objectives, and expected outcomes.

Observation and Modification:

For the duration of Itravil therapy, regular monitoring is essential to guaranteeing both safety and efficacy. Healthcare professionals should evaluate the patient's cardiovascular health, weight loss progress, and any possible side effects. Based on these evaluations, dosage modifications might be required, carefully considering how to strike a balance between reaching weight loss objectives and lowering hazards.

If there is not enough of a response or if side effects start to appear, medical professionals might change the dosage, temporarily stop the treatment, or look into other weight-management options. Itravil therapy's customized nature necessitates constant attention to detail and a proactive approach to modifying the treatment plan in response to the patient's changing needs.

Itravil's dosage and administration reflect the careful balancing act between safety concerns and therapeutic efficacy. Effective incorporation of Itravil into weight control regimens is facilitated by the customized approach to dosage determination, meticulous assessment of patient attributes, and cooperative treatment planning.

Healthcare providers act as mentors and collaborators with their patients as they work to achieve healthier body weights, assisting them as they negotiate the challenges of prescription Itravil. Itravil can play a vital part in the all-encompassing approach to weight management with careful adherence to dosing rules, clear patient communication, and continuous monitoring.

CONTRAINDICATIONS

A critical component of ethical medicine is the definition of contraindications, which helps medical professionals recognize situations in which a patient's use of a specific prescription is either expressly forbidden or fraught with danger. To protect patient safety and direct treatment choices, a thorough knowledge of contraindications is essential when it comes to Itravil, a drug intended for weight control. This in-depth investigation will focus on the cases when Itravil should not be used, as well as those that call for extreme caution and careful thought.

COMPLETE RESTRICTIONS:

Heart-related Conditions:

People who have a history of cardiovascular conditions, such as uncontrolled hypertension, heart failure, arrhythmias, or coronary artery disease, should not take iretavil.
Itravil's sympathomimetic effects, which raise blood pressure and heart rate, provide a serious risk to people with weak cardiovascular systems.

Overactive thyroid function:

People who have hyperthyroidism, a disorder marked by an overactive thyroid gland, are thought to be more susceptible to negative cardiovascular outcomes.
Itravil's stimulant qualities may make hyperthyroidism symptoms worse, thus it's important to use cautious in this demographic.
glaucoma
For those suffering with narrow-angle glaucoma, which is characterized by elevated intraocular pressure, it is not recommended to use istravil.
Itravil's sympathomimetic actions have the potential to exacerbate glaucoma and jeopardize eye health.

Substance Abuse History:

Dependency is more likely to develop in people with a history of substance usage, especially with stimulant or anorexigenic substances.
Itravil is not recommended for people with a history of drug use disorders due to the possibility of misuse and dependence.

Getting pregnant and nursing:

Due to insufficient safety information during pregnancy and the possibility of the medication leaking into breast milk, it is not recommended for use by women who are pregnant or nursing.
Itravil is an unacceptable choice in these populations since the dangers to the growing fetus and the infant outweigh any potential advantages.

Situations Needing Caution:

Even if the preceding list of contraindications is exhaustive, there are some circumstances that call for caution and cautious consideration before using Itravil. While using Itravil may not always be prohibited by these conditions, healthcare professionals should carefully monitor patients and balance any possible hazards against any benefits.

Impairment of Renal Function:

Because renal insufficiency may alter drug metabolism and elimination, dose modifications may be necessary for these individuals.

It is recommended to closely monitor renal function and to modify the dosage in accordance with the severity of impairment.

The Past of Mental Illnesses:

Those who have already had mental health issues, such as anxiety or depression, may be more vulnerable to Itravil's mood-altering effects.
Patients should exercise caution and have their moods observed for any changes or worsening of mental disorders.

Senior Citizens:

Elderly people might need smaller starting doses since they may be more vulnerable to negative cardiovascular consequences.
In this population, it is important to monitor for any side effects, particularly cardiovascular abnormalities.

Mellitus diabetes:

Blood glucose levels in people with diabetes mellitus may fluctuate while using Itravil medication.
It can be essential to regularly check blood glucose levels and modify anti-diabetic drug dosages.

The past of seizures:

People who have a history of seizures should exercise caution when using Itravil since it may lower the threshold for seizures.
It is important to thoroughly evaluate the risk-benefit balance and keep an eye out for any indications that a patient may be more susceptible to seizures.

Relationships with Substances That Are Contraindicated:

Itravil may interact with several drugs and substances, causing side effects or escalating its effects. It is essential to comprehend these relationships in order to avoid possibly dangerous outcomes. Among the noteworthy exchanges are:

- MAOIs, or monoamine oxidase inhibitors: Because of the possibility of a hypertensive crisis, using Itravil with MAOIs at the same time is not recommended.
  To reduce this risk, a long enough washout interval between MAOIs and Itravil is necessary.
- Additional Sympathomimetic Drugs: When Itravil is taken with other sympathomimetic drugs, the effects on the heart could get worse.
- Itravil must be prescribed with caution and under close observation when combined with other sympathomimetic medications.

In summary, healthcare professionals who are tasked with writing prescriptions for Itravil must possess a thorough grasp of the contraindications related to this medicine. Absolute contraindications, like pregnancy and cardiovascular conditions, necessitate careful adherence to prescription recommendations in order to protect patient safety.

Conditions that call for caution also emphasize the necessity of a complete patient assessment and continuing observation in order to identify and control any hazards. Interactions with substances that are contraindicated highlight how crucial thorough medication evaluations and provider communication are to averting unfavorable consequences.

Healthcare practitioners may traverse the intricacies of contraindications and ensure that Itravil is provided prudently and safely in the context of each patient's needs and health status by incorporating this knowledge into their clinical decision-making.

ADVERSE REACTIONS

Responsible medication must include both the detection and treatment of adverse effects. Itravil is a drug intended to help with weight management, however it has a number of possible side effects. This thorough investigation will examine the various side effects associated with Itravil, including physiologic, psychological, and systemic impacts. In order to protect patients and make wise decisions during weight control therapy, healthcare professionals must be aware of these undesirable responses.

TYPICAL ADVERSE OUTCOMES:

Effects on the Heart:

The most common adverse reactions that are noticed are cardiovascular ones, such as raised blood pressure and heart rate.

The sympathomimetic qualities of Itravil cause increased cardiovascular activity by imitating the functions of the sympathetic nervous system.

Sleeplessness:

Itravil's stimulant qualities could be a factor in problems falling or staying asleep.
To reduce the chance of sleeplessness, patients should be instructed to take their prescription earlier in the day.

Parched Mouth:

Dry mouth is a frequent adverse effect of sympathomimetic drugs, and it can happen with Itravil.
It is advised to practice proper dental hygiene and stay hydrated in order to reduce this sensation.

Disorders of the Gastrointestines:

Adverse reactions involving the digestive system, like nausea, constipation, or diarrhea, can happen.
These symptoms can be controlled by varying when Itravil is administered in relation to meals and making sure you're getting enough fluids.

Feeling uneasy and restless:

Some people may become more tense or restless, which is indicative of Itravil's stimulant properties. Encouraging patients to identify and manage these feelings is crucial for maintaining compliance with treatment as a whole.

LESS FREQUENT ADVERSE EVENTS:

Mood Shifts:

Itravil users may experience mood swings, such as heightened emotional reactivity, anxiety, or irritation.
Healthcare professionals should keep an eye out for these changes and, if necessary, adjust dosages or use different strategies.

Tachycardia:

Apart from the typical cardiovascular consequences, tachycardia a condition marked by an unusually high heart rate may occur in certain people.

Frequent heart rate monitoring is essential, and if tachycardia persists, dose modifications can be needed.

Headache:

One less prevalent side effect linked to Itravil is headache.
Patients should be encouraged to report severe or ongoing headaches, and medical professionals should look into other possibilities for therapy if needed.

Trembling:

Some people may experience tremors after taking sympathomimetic drugs like Itravil.
It's crucial to keep an eye out for tremors that appear or get worse, especially in patients who already have tremor-related illnesses.

Feeling lightheaded:

It is possible to feel lightheaded or dizzy, especially in the early stages of treatment.

Potential postural alterations and the significance of slowly rising from a seated or sleeping position should be explained to patients.

SEVERE ADVERSE EVENTS:

- High blood pressure: Because of the way that Itravil affects blood pressure, people who already have hypertension may develop hypertension.
- It's important to regularly check blood pressure, and if it stays high for an extended period of time, Itravil may need to be stopped.
- Events Related to the Heart: Serious cardiovascular problems like myocardial infarction or stroke might happen in rare cases.
- Patients with a history of cardiovascular illness should not use Itravil, and medical professionals should be on the lookout for any warning indications of a serious cardiovascular event.
- Psychological Impacts: There have been reports of severe psychiatric side effects,

including as psychosis, hallucinations, and extreme agitation.

- People who have a history of mental illnesses should be continuously watched, and if they exhibit serious mental symptoms, they should get help right away.
- Convulsions: Itravil usage has the potential to cause seizures by lowering the seizure threshold.
- Itravil may need to be avoided in patients who have a history of seizures or other risk conditions; these patients should be thoroughly assessed.
- Reactions Allergic to: Allergy reactions can cause swelling, irritation, or skin rashes, albeit they are uncommon.
- If a patient exhibits symptoms that could indicate an allergic response, they should be advised to get medical help right away.

CONTROLLING ADVERSE REACTIONS:

- Frequent Observation: It is essential to regularly monitor vital indicators, such as blood pressure and heart rate, in order to identify and treat cardiovascular consequences.

Frequent follow-up sessions offer the chance to evaluate the status of weight loss and spot any new adverse events.

- Patient Instruction: When it comes to controlling adverse reactions, patient education is crucial. Patients are more likely to stick to treatment programs when there is clear communication regarding possible side effects, how long they should last, and coping mechanisms.

  Proactive management is enhanced by giving patients the tools they need to identify and promptly report adverse effects.

- Dosage modifications: Dosage changes may be taken into consideration to maximize the risk-benefit profile in cases of mild adverse effects.

  Reducing the amount or adjusting the timing of the dose could help lessen some adverse effects.

- Therapy Termination: Itravil therapy may have to be stopped if side effects become severe or persistent.

A thorough evaluation of the patient's general health and the trade-off between the possible hazards and therapeutic advantages should inform the decision to stop.

- Alternative Medical Interventions: When contraindications occur or bad responses become intolerable, medical professionals may look into alternate weight-management techniques.

  A smooth transition to an alternate strategy depends on collaborative decision-making with the patient.

Healthcare professionals providing weight management therapy must have a thorough grasp of the side effects linked to Itravil. Understanding the many physiological, psychological, and systemic impacts makes proactive management possible and improves Itravil's overall safety and effectiveness.

Healthcare practitioners are capable of navigating the complexity of adverse responses by means of vigilant monitoring, patient education, and strategic interventions. This approach guarantees that Itravil is used prudently and that the well-being of individuals on weight control journeys is given priority.

DRUG INTERACTIONS

Any medication's potential for drug interactions must be taken into account for safe and efficient use. The weight-management drug Itravil is not immune to the intricate web of interactions that can arise while taking various medications at the same time. This thorough investigation will cover both pharmacokinetic and pharmacodynamic medication interactions related to Itravil, in addition to offering insights into the mechanisms, clinical consequences, and management methods.

DRUG-COOPERATIVE INTERACTIONS:

- CYP3A4 Inhibitors: The main enzyme system that breaks down itravil is cytochrome P450, namely CYP3A4. Elevated blood concentrations of Itravil may occur from co-administration with potent CYP3A4 inhibitors such ritonavir or ketoconazole.
- Clinical Implications: Higher Itravil concentrations may intensify its effects and raise the possibility of negative side effects. In such circumstances, dose modifications or

other weight-management techniques might be taken into consideration.

- CYP2D6 Inhibitors: CYP2D6 inhibitors, like paroxetine or fluoxetine, may affect how Itravil is metabolized. Clobenzorex, the active ingredient in Itravil, is converted to amphetamine by CYP2D6.

- Clinical Implications: A lower efficacy could arise from a reduced conversion of clobenzorex to amphetamine. It could be necessary to keep an eye out for decreased weight loss effects and think about switching to another drug.

- CYP2B6 Triggers: Itravil's metabolism may be improved by medications that increase CYP2B6, such as rifampin or efavirenz, which may lower the drug's plasma level.

- Clinical Implications: Itravil's effectiveness may be hampered by lower levels. Vigilant observation and perhaps modifications to dosage or substitute tactics would be required.

- Agents for Gastrointestinal Alkalization: Itravil absorption may change if gastrointestinal alkalizing medications, such as proton pump inhibitors, are used concurrently.

- Clinical Implications: A decrease in effectiveness could result from a reduction in absorption. This interaction might be lessened if Itravil and alkalizing drugs are administered separately.

PHARMACODYNAMIC CONCURRENT EVENTS:

- Agents that Sympathomimetic: Additive cardiovascular effects may result with the concurrent use of other sympathomimetic drugs, such as decongestants or stimulant medicines.
- Clinical Implications: Caution is advised due to the potential dangers associated with elevated blood pressure and heart rate. It could be required to monitor for cardiovascular effects and take dose adjustments into consideration.
- Depression-fighting drugs: Itravil interactions with selective serotonin reuptake inhibitors (SSRIs) and serotonin-norepinephrine

reuptake inhibitors (SNRIs) may raise the risk of serotonin syndrome.

- Clinical Implications: It is important to keep an eye out for signs of serotonin syndrome, including agitation, hyperreflexia, and fever. Alternative drugs or dose modifications might be taken into consideration.
- Drugs that lower blood pressure: The sympathomimetic properties of Itravil may negate the antihypertensive effects of beta- or alpha-blockers.
- Clinical Implications: To keep blood pressure within goal limits, antihypertensive medication changes may be required in addition to close monitoring of blood pressure.
- MAOIs: Because of the possibility of a hypertensive crisis, using Itravil and monoamine oxidase inhibitors (MAOIs) at the same time is not advised.
- Clinical Implications: In order to reduce the risk of hypertensive crisis, there must be a sufficient washout period between MAOIs and Itravil.
- Anti-serotonergic Drugs: Serotonin syndrome risk may rise if Itravil is used with other

serotonergic drugs, like tramadol or other migraine medicines.

- Clinical Implications: It is important to keep an eye out for serotonin syndrome signs. To reduce this risk, different pharmaceutical options or dose modifications may be taken into consideration.

TECHNIQUES OF MANAGEMENT:

Thorough Review of Medication:

To find any interactions, a complete examination of the patient's prescription, over-the-counter, and herbal product list is necessary.

- Clinical Implications: By doing routine drug evaluations, medical professionals can avoid unfavorable outcomes, modify treatment strategies, and make educated decisions.
- Patient Instruction:It is essential to educate patients on the significance of telling healthcare professionals about all medications, even over-the-counter drugs.
- Clinical Implications: Accurate medication histories are improved by improved communication, which helps medical

professionals foresee and efficiently handle possible interactions.

- Dosage modifications: Dosage modifications may be taken into consideration when interactions are found in order to maximize therapeutic benefits and reduce hazards.
- Clinical Implications: Clinical surveillance and a careful evaluation of the ratio between efficacy and possible side effects should serve as a guide for dose adjustments.
- Alternative Medical Interventions: Alternative approaches to weight management or drugs with a better interaction profile may be taken into consideration when substantial interactions present obstacles to safe and successful therapy.
- Clinical Implications: The features, preferences, and overall therapeutic objectives of each patient should be taken into consideration while choosing alternative therapies.
- Monitoring Specifics: When interacting drugs are present, it is imperative to regularly evaluate clinical parameters such as blood

pressure, heart rate, and any potential signs of harmful effects.

- Clinical Implications: Proactive intervention and treatment plan modification are made possible by early detection of changes in vital signs or symptoms.

Handling medication interactions with Itravil requires a comprehensive strategy that incorporates both pharmacokinetic and pharmacodynamic aspects. In order to guarantee the safe and efficient use of Itravil in the context of weight control, healthcare providers must successfully negotiate the complex web of interactions.

Healthcare providers can reduce the chances of drug interactions by carefully reviewing medications, educating patients, making judicious dose adjustments, and taking alternative therapy into account. In the dynamic field of weight management, this proactive and customized approach adds to the overall safety and efficacy of Itravil therapy.

PRECAUTIONS AND WARNINGS

To guarantee the safe and efficient use of Itravil, one must have a thorough awareness of the cautions and warnings related to its administration. Itravil is a weight-management medicine that has a number of adverse effect considerations that are meant to be minimized and therapeutic benefits maximized. This comprehensive analysis will examine the several safety measures and alerts related to Itravil, including patient selection, parameter monitoring, and particular demographics that need extra care.

SELECTION AND EVALUATION OF PATIENTS:

Heart Health:

It is critical to thoroughly evaluate cardiovascular health before starting Itravil medication. A higher risk may apply to people having a history of cardiovascular conditions, such as uncontrolled hypertension, heart failure, arrhythmias, or coronary artery disease.

- Clinical Implications: It's critical to closely monitor cardiovascular indicators like blood pressure and heart rate. It can be appropriate to take into account different weight-management techniques for those who have serious cardiovascular issues.

High blood pressure:

Before beginning Itravil, people with pre-existing hypertension should have a thorough evaluation. High blood pressure may result from the medication's sympathomimetic effects.

- Clinical Implications: To keep blood pressure within goal ranges, regular blood pressure monitoring may be required, along with consideration of antihypertensive drugs or dose modifications.

Substance Abuse History:

Dependency may be more likely among people with a history of substance addiction, particularly with stimulant or anorexigenic substances.

- Clinical Implications: Selecting patients carefully requires determining whether or not they have a history of misuse or dependence. For those with a history of substance addiction, other therapy may be taken into consideration, and close observation for indications of misuse or dependence is necessary.

Psychiatric Conditions:

Those who have already had mental health issues such as anxiety, depression, or bipolar disorder may be especially vulnerable to Itravil's mood-altering effects.

- Clinical Implications: Care should be taken, and mood swings or an aggravation of mental disorders should be regularly observed. Working together with mental health specialists could be advantageous.

Senior Citizens:

The pharmacokinetics of Itravil may be impacted by age-related changes in drug metabolism, and elderly people may be more vulnerable to harmful cardiovascular consequences.

- Clinical Implications: In the elderly population, lower starting dosages and close observation for side effects are advised. All possible drug interactions should be carefully considered.

MONITORING SPECIFICS:

Heart-Risk Assessment:

Throughout the course of Itravil therapy, regular monitoring of cardiovascular indicators, such as blood pressure and heart rate, is essential.
Clinical Implications: Proactive intervention and plan modification to reduce cardiovascular risks are made possible by early identification of changes in vital signs.

Progress in Losing Weight:

Assessing weight reduction progress continuously is essential to figuring out how successful Itravil medication is.

- Clinical Implications: Keeping an eye on weight loss patterns enables medical professionals to make well-informed judgments on the continuation of therapy and may direct modifications to the treatment regimen.

Psychological Surveillance:

Regular psychiatric monitoring is recommended for those with a history of mental problems in order to identify any changes in mood or worsening of symptoms.

- Clinical Implications: When there are notable psychiatric effects, early intervention and consultation with mental health specialists may be required.

Renal Function:

Because renal insufficiency may alter drug metabolism and elimination, dosage modifications may be necessary for these patients.

- Clinical Implications: It is recommended to regularly check renal function and to modify dosage in accordance with the severity of impairment.

Levels of blood glucose:

Since Itravil may affect glucose metabolism, those with diabetes mellitus should have their blood glucose levels checked on a regular basis.

- Clinical Implications: Depending on changes in blood glucose levels, antidiabetic medication adjustments may be required.

PARTICULAR POPULATIONS:

Getting pregnant and nursing:

Due to insufficient safety information during pregnancy and the possibility of the medication leaking into breast milk, it is not recommended for use by women who are pregnant or nursing.

- Clinical Implications: Before beginning Itravil medication, a pregnancy test and advice on safe contraception are necessary. During treatment, breastfeeding should be avoided.

Children's Population:

Itravil's safety and effectiveness in pediatric populations are unknown, and using it in those less than 18 is typically not advised.

- Clinical Implications: For juvenile patients, alternative weight control techniques should be taken into account, and the advantages and disadvantages of pharmacological therapies in this population should be carefully evaluated.

Senior Citizenry:

The pharmacokinetics of Itravil may be impacted by age-related changes in drug metabolism, and elderly people may be more vulnerable to harmful cardiovascular consequences.

- Clinical Implications: In the senior population, it may be recommended to investigate other weight management measures, monitor closely, and start with lower beginning dosages.

Hepatic or Renal Impairment:

Dosage adjustments may be necessary for patients with renal or hepatic impairment because of possible variations in medication metabolism and elimination.

- Clinical Implications: Dosage should be modified in accordance with the degree of impairment, and regular monitoring of liver and kidney function is advised.

PRECAUTIONS TO TAKE DURING THERAPY:

Patient Instruction:

It is crucial to educate patients on the significance of adhering to recommended dosages, possible adverse effects, and the necessity of scheduling frequent follow-up appointments.

- Clinical Implications: Giving patients information improves treatment compliance and makes it possible to identify and report side effects early on.

Modifications to Diet and Lifestyle:

Itravil therapy should include a strong emphasis on the value of dietary and lifestyle modifications, such as a balanced diet and increased physical exercise.

- Clinical Implications: The chance of long-term weight loss and general well-being is increased when pharmaceutical intervention and lifestyle changes are combined.

Gradual Stoppage:

If you stop taking Itravil suddenly, you can have withdrawal symptoms. Dosage reduction gradually might be taken into consideration.

- Clinical Implications: A well-thought-out cessation approach helps minimize withdrawal symptoms, and collaborative decision-making with the patient is essential.:

The cautions and warnings related to Itravil highlight the significance of thorough patient assessment, close observation, and cooperative decision-making between patients and healthcare professionals. Healthcare practitioners can maximize the safety and efficacy of Itravil therapy in the dynamic setting of weight management by negotiating the intricacies of patient selection, monitoring parameters, and concerns for particular populations.

OVERDOSAGE

Any medication has the potential to be overdosed, hence it is important to fully comprehend the pharmacology, clinical symptoms, and management techniques. The medicine Itravil, which is intended to help regulate weight, is not immune to overdosage risks. The present investigation aims to examine all facets of Itravil overdosage, including the drug's pharmacokinetics, overdose symptoms, and suitable therapeutic approaches to minimize hazards and guarantee patient well-being.

Itravil pharmacokinetics:

Determining the possible effects of overdosage requires an understanding of Itravil's pharmacokinetics. Clobenzorex hydrochloride, an agent that functions as a sympathomimetic, is the active component of Itravil. When clobenzorex is broken down, amphetamine, a substance that stimulates the central nervous system, is produced.

Take-up:

Following oral dosing, itravil is absorbed from the gastrointestinal system.
After consumption, peak plasma concentrations usually occur a few hours later.

The metabolism:

Clobenzorex is metabolized in the liver, mostly by the cytochrome P450 enzyme system, in which CYP3A4 is an important participant.
Amphetamine is produced through metabolism and adds to Itravil's overall pharmacological effects.

Removal:

Clobenzorex has a brief elimination half-life and is mostly eliminated through the urine.
The prolonged persistence of pharmacological effects is partly attributed to the synthesis of amphetamine, which has a longer elimination half-life.

Overdosage Clinical Manifestations:

A variety of clinical symptoms may arise from an Itravil overdose, which is indicative of the stimulant characteristics of clobenzorex and its metabolite amphetamine. The quantity consumed as well as unique patient characteristics can affect how severe the symptoms are.

Effects on the Heart:

The most common cardiovascular symptoms of an Itravil overdose are tachycardia, palpitations, and increased blood pressure.
More serious cardiovascular problems, such as arrhythmias, myocardial infarction, or stroke, may develop in severe situations.

Stimulation of the central nervous system:

A central nervous system that is overstimulated may cause anxiety, restlessness, agitation, and sleeplessness.
Certain people may experience seizures, particularly those who have a history of seizure disorders or a propensity to them.

Disorders of the Gastrointestines:

When someone takes too much Itravil, they may experience nausea, vomiting, and stomach pain.
Electrolyte imbalances and dehydration can be exacerbated by gastrointestinal symptoms.

Psychological Impacts:

Severe overdosage may cause exaggeration of psychiatric consequences, such as hallucinations, psychosis, and extreme agitation.
People who already suffer from mental illnesses could be more vulnerable to these consequences.

Overheating:

Itravil's sympathomimetic actions may cause hyperthermia, or elevated body temperature.
Serious repercussions from extreme heat include organ damage and multiple organ failure.

Controlling Itravil Overdosage:

Itravil overdose is managed in a complex way that includes supportive care, symptomatic treatment, and ways to improve drug excretion. Reducing medication absorption, symptom relief, and avoiding or controlling problems are the objectives of management.

Charcoal that has been activated:

To stop Itravil from being absorbed further, activated charcoal may be administered in the initial hours following consumption.
Early initiation of this intervention is optimal for its effectiveness, and it can be especially helpful in cases of recent overdose.

Gastric Rinse:

When there has been a substantial overdose, especially if the consumption happened quickly, stomach pumping, or gastric lavage, may be advised.
This process, which can be carried out under medical supervision, aids in getting the medication out of the stomach.

Assistive Healthcare:

It is crucial to provide supportive care, which entails keeping an eye on vital signs, staying well-hydrated, and handling problems as they appear.
Cardiovascular monitoring is essential, and it could be necessary to take measures to stabilize heart rate and blood pressure.

Benzodiazepines:

Benzodiazepines can be used to treat agitation, seizures, and stimulation of the central nervous system.
These medications can aid in the management of symptoms and stop more issues brought on by high CNS activity.

Antipyretics:

Antipyretic drugs, including acetaminophen, may be used to reduce body temperature in cases of hyperthermia.
In addition, cooling techniques like tepid sponge bathing can be used to treat hyperthermia.

Management of Fluid and Electrolyte:

Electrolyte imbalances and dehydration may be caused by gastrointestinal disorders. Maintaining hydration and reestablishing electrolyte balance may require intravenous fluid administration.
We're keeping an eye out for electrolyte imbalances and indicators of dehydration.

Interventions for Cardiovascular Disease:

Interventions to treat arrhythmias and regulate blood pressure may be required in cases of significant cardiovascular consequences.
In cases of severe cardiovascular impairment, consultation with a cardiologist or critical care specialist may be necessary.

Mental Health Consultation:

For assessment and treatment, severe mental side effects including psychosis or hallucinations may call for contact with a psychiatric professional.
People with pre-existing mental illnesses could need continuous mental health treatment.

Hemodialysis:

In cases of severe overdosage, particularly if there is evidence of renal impairment, hemodialysis may be considered.
Hemodialysis can improve the drug's and its metabolites' excretion from the body.

OBSERVATION AND SUCCESSION:

Constant Observation:

It is imperative to maintain constant observation of vital indicators, such as blood pressure, temperature, and heart rate, while an overdose is acute.
Frequent clinical evaluations aid in determining the success of therapies and provide direction for future care.

Monitoring of an electrocardiogram (ECG):

Frequent or continuous ECG monitoring is essential for identifying and treating any conduction anomalies or arrhythmias.
In situations where there are cardiovascular issues, this surveillance is very crucial.

Analysis of Serial Blood Gases:

To evaluate the state of oxygenation and the acid-base balance, serial blood gas analysis may be carried out.
It's critical to keep an eye out for metabolic acidosis, particularly in cases of severe overdosage.

Monitoring of Renal Function:

It is crucial to monitor renal function, including blood urea nitrogen (BUN) and serum creatinine, particularly if hemodialysis is being considered.
The overall evaluation includes making sure the urine production is sufficient.

Psychiatric Aftercare:

Psychiatric follow-up may be beneficial for people who suffer from severe mental side effects in order to monitor for persistent symptoms and administer the necessary treatments.
In order to manage complex patients, collaboration between medical and psychiatric doctors is crucial.

Managing an overdose of Itravil necessitates a thorough and organized strategy that takes into account the drug's pharmacokinetics, overdose symptoms, and suitable risk-reduction measures. Overdose management is more successful overall when supportive care, symptomatic treatment, and steps to improve drug elimination are started on time.

Healthcare professionals should have the skills and tools necessary to identify and appropriately treat Itravil overdose, with an emphasis on reducing side effects and safeguarding the health of those who may be at risk. Managing complicated cases of Itravil overdosage may need collaboration across multiple medical specialties, including as emergency medicine, cardiology, psychiatry, and nephrology.

CLINICAL PHARMACOLOGY

The weight-management drug Itravil has a unique clinical pharmacology profile that is important to both its therapeutic efficacy and possible adverse effects. This thorough investigation will cover several facets of Itravil's clinical pharmacology, including its pharmacodynamics, pharmacokinetics, and mechanism of action, as well as how these elements affect the drug's overall safety and efficacy.

PHARMACODYNAMICS:

Property Sympathomimetic:

Itravil mimics the functions of the sympathetic nervous system in order to achieve its pharmacological effects. This is known as sympathomimetic activity.

- Clinical Implications: Heart rate, blood pressure, and thermogenesis are all boosted by sympathomimetic effects. These support the medication's ability to decrease appetite and promote weight loss.

Stimulation of the central nervous system:

Itravil stimulates the central nervous system by releasing neurotransmitters including dopamine and norepinephrine.

- Clinical Implications: Enhanced activity of the central nervous system is linked to elevated energy levels generally, reduced weariness, and enhanced attentiveness. The patient's capacity to stick to dietary and lifestyle changes may be impacted by these impacts.

Suppression of Appetite:

Itravil suppresses appetite by acting on the brain's satiety centers through sympathomimetic effects.
Clinical Implications: Eating less food results in a negative energy balance, which encourages weight loss. The consequences of lowering appetite, however, may differ from person to person.

Effects of Thermogen:

Itravil's sympathomimetic properties promote thermogenesis, the body's process of producing heat.

- Clinical Implications: Itravil's effects on weight loss are supported by increased thermogenesis, which increases total energy expenditure.

PHARMACOKINETICS:

Take-up:

When taken orally, Itravil's active component, clobenzorex, is absorbed through the digestive system.

- Clinical Implications: Itravil's overall bioavailability and rate of action are influenced by the degree and pace of absorption.

The metabolism:

Clobenzorex is metabolized in the liver, mostly by the cytochrome P450 enzyme system, in which CYP3A4 is an important participant.

- Clinical Implications: Itravil's pharmacological actions are partially attributed to amphetamine, an active metabolite formed by metabolism.

Metabolism may be impacted by CYP3A4-affecting genetic and pharmacological interactions.

Distribution:

Plasma proteins are involved in the dispersion of Itravil and its metabolites; amphetamine acts more slowly.

- Clinical Implications: Distribution affects the possibility of accumulation and the length of therapeutic benefits, particularly with long-term treatment.

Removal:

Urine is the main organ where clobenzorex and its metabolites are eliminated.

- Clinical Implications: Because renal function affects how quickly Itravil is eliminated, those with renal impairment may require dose modifications.

Half-Life:

Clobenzorex has a short half-life for elimination, whereas amphetamine has a longer half-life and helps to prolong the effects of Itravil.

- Clinical Implications: The duration of effect overall and the frequency of dose are influenced by the pharmacokinetic profile.

ACTION MECHANISM:

Effects of Dopamine and Noradrenergic Reactions:

Enhancement of dopaminergic and noradrenergic neurotransmission in the central nervous system is the mechanism of action of istravil.

- Clinical Implications: Elevated arousal, higher energy expenditure, and hunger suppression are caused by elevated synaptic levels of dopamine and norepinephrine.

Centers for Appetite Control:

Itravil's sympathomimetic effects alter the hypothalamic centers responsible for controlling hunger.

- Clinical Implications: Appetite center regulation helps people stick to diets low in calories by reducing sensations of hunger.

Increasing Thermogenesis:

Itravil activates beta-adrenergic receptors, which in turn promotes thermogenesis.

- Clinical Implications: Weight loss is facilitated by increased thermogenesis, which encourages the use of stored fat as fuel.

Effects on the Periphery:

Peripheral tissues are affected by the sympathomimetic effects, which also affect energy consumption and metabolic rate.

- Clinical Implications: Itravil's peripheral effects affect weight loss outcomes by contributing to its total metabolic effects.

VARIABILITY IN REACTION:

Individual Variations

Genetic variances, changes in drug metabolism, and variations in the sensitivity of neurotransmitter receptors can all affect an individual's reaction to Itravil.

- Clinical Implications: Customizing treatment regimens based on the unique needs of each patient may maximize therapeutic results and reduce the possibility of side effects.

Dependency and Tolerance:

When using sympathomimetic drugs for an extended period of time, such as Itravil, tolerance may develop, necessitating dose increases to maintain effects.

- Clinical Implications: It is imperative to regularly check for the development of dependence and tolerance. When stopping therapy, a gradual taper may be required.

CLINICAL PERFORMANCE:

Advantages of Losing Weight:

Itravil's main clinical benefit is its ability to suppress appetite, enhance energy expenditure, and modulate central nervous system activity in order to facilitate weight loss.

- Clinical Implications: When Itravil is used in conjunction with other comprehensive strategies such as dietary adjustments and increased physical activity, the advantages of weight loss are most noticeable.

Maintaining Weight Loss:

Itravil is frequently prescribed for a brief period of time to help people lose weight, with the goal of encouraging long-term lifestyle changes that will help them maintain their weight.

- Clinical Implications: In addition to medication intervention, healthcare personnel are essential in teaching patients the value of lifestyle adjustments.

Handling Comorbidities:

Itravil-acquired weight loss may help address comorbid diseases like insulin resistance, dyslipidemia, and hypertension that are linked to obesity.

- Clinical Implications: An essential component of Itravil therapy's overall health benefits is the monitoring and management of comorbidities connected to obesity.

NEGATIVE IMPACTS:

Effects on the Heart:

Itravil frequently causes adverse cardiovascular symptoms, such as palpitations, raised blood pressure, and an accelerated heartbeat.

- Clinical Implications: Patients with pre-existing cardiovascular problems should exercise caution and should undergo regular cardiovascular monitoring.

Effects on the Central Nervous System:

Itravil side effects that typically affect the central nervous system include anxiety, restlessness, and insomnia.

- Clinical Implications: Managing effects on the central nervous system may require varying dosages, scheduling dosages optimally, or exploring alternate therapies.

Disorders of the Gastrointestines:

Itravil frequently causes gastrointestinal side effects, including as nausea, constipation, and dry mouth.

- Clinical Implications: Treatment adherence is influenced by symptomatic management and patient education regarding the mitigation of gastrointestinal problems.

Psychological Impacts:

When using Itravil, psychiatric side effects such as agitation, mood swings, and, in rare cases, hallucinations, may manifest.

- Clinical Implications: It's important to keep an eye out for any psychiatric side effects, particularly in people who already have mental illnesses.

Symptoms of Withdrawal:

Itravil withdrawal symptoms, including as lethargy, depression, and appetite changes, might occur with an abrupt stop.

- Clinical Implications: Patients should be educated about the discontinuation process and their dosage should be tapered gradually to reduce the severity of withdrawal symptoms.

INTERACTIONS BETWEEN DRUGS:

Interactions of CYP3A4:

Itravil is metabolized by CYP3A4, and interactions between this enzyme's inducers and inhibitors can affect the amount of the drug in the body.

- Clinical Implications: Dosage adjustments may be required when Itravil is taken with medications that interfere with CYP3A4 activity.

Anti-serotonergic Drugs:

Serotonin syndrome risk may rise if Itravil is used concurrently with other serotonergic drugs.

- Clinical Implications: When taking Itravil alongside other drugs that affect serotonin levels, caution and close observation are necessary.

Drugs that lower blood pressure:

The sympathomimetic effects of Itravil may negate the hypotensive effects of beta-blockers and other medicines.

- Clinical Implications: It may be required to modify antihypertensive drug dosages and perform routine blood pressure monitoring.

Pharmacodynamics, pharmacokinetics, and mechanisms of action are intricately intertwined in the clinical pharmacology of Itravil. Healthcare professionals must comprehend these factors in order to maximize Itravil's benefits while lowering any risks or negative side effects. In the ever-changing field of weight management, tailored treatment regimens, consistent observation, and patient education all play a part in the overall effectiveness of Itravil therapy.

HOW SUPPLIED/STORAGE AND HANDLING

To guarantee the medicine's efficacy and safety, healthcare professionals, pharmacists, and patients must have access to information about how a medication is provided, kept, and handled. This thorough investigation will include the specifics of Itravil's delivery, suggested storage settings, and handling instructions to preserve the drug's stability and purity.

Forms of Dosage:

Oral dose forms like tablets or capsules are frequently offered for Itravil.

- Clinical Implications: Depending on the pharmaceutical manufacturer, the precise dose form may change. In order to administer the right formulation, healthcare professionals should be aware of the various forms that are available.

Advantages:

To facilitate customized treatment strategies, Itravil may be provided in varying strengths.

- Clinical Implications: When prescribing Itravil, prescribers should indicate the desired strength while considering the patient's needs and the suggested dosage for weight control.

Packaging:

Usually, Itravil comes in bottles or blister packs, each of which holds a certain number of pills or capsules.

- Clinical Implications: To guarantee the integrity of the medicine, pharmacists should inspect the packaging for evidence of tampering or damage prior to administering the medication.

Patient Information Pamphlet:

A patient information sheet that contains vital information about Itravil, such as indications, dose guidelines, possible side effects, and safety data, is included with each package of the drug.

- Clinical Implications: Physicians should advise patients to read the patient information booklet carefully and to contact them with any queries or concerns.

Requirements for Prescription:

Itravil is usually only available with a prescription, and medical professionals should abide by regional laws and prescribing policies.

- Clinical Implications: Doctors need to provide patients precise directions regarding dosage, length of treatment, and any unique needs.

CONDITIONS OF STORAGE:

Warmth:

It is recommended that Itravil be kept in a controlled room temperature range of 20 to 25 degrees Celsius (68 to 77 degrees Fahrenheit).

- Clinical Implications: Keeping medication stored within the suggested temperature range contributes to its stability and effectiveness.

Avoiding exposure to very high or low temperatures is advised.

Defense Against Light:

Itravil needs to be shielded from light, and the materials used for packaging need to be sufficiently resistant to light.

- Clinical Implications: The medication's active components may deteriorate if exposed to light. It is therefore advised to store Itravil in its original packing or in a container that is resistant to light.

Considering Moisture:

It is recommended to store Itravil in a dry area with precautions taken to avoid moisture exposure.

- Clinical Implications: The stability of the medication may be jeopardized by moisture, which could result in modifications to its chemical and physical composition. It is imperative to store items away from moist surroundings.

Containers Resistant to Children:

Child-resistant elements are frequently included in Itravil packaging to improve safety, particularly in homes with small children.

- Clinical Implications: Pharmacists should advise patients to keep drugs out of the reach of children and supply Itravil in child-resistant containers.

Particular Storage Guidelines:

On the box or in the prescribed literature, the manufacturer might include detailed storage instructions.

- Clinical Implications: In order to maintain the stability of the medication, healthcare professionals, pharmacists, and patients should follow any special storage guidelines supplied by the manufacturer.

GUIDELINES FOR HANDLING:

Healthcare Professionals' Dispensing:

When giving patients Itravil, medical personnel including pharmacists should adhere to established guidelines.

- Clinical Implications: Ensuring precise dispensing, giving patients clear instructions, and attending to any queries or concerns all help to ensure that medications are used safely.

Patient Instruction Regarding Storage:

Itravil should be stored correctly; patients should be made aware of this, stressing the need to keep the drug out of direct sunlight and in a cold, dry location.

- Clinical Implications: In order to preserve the safety and efficacy of the drug, patients must follow to storage standards. Having more knowledge can assist avoid storage-related problems.

Preventing Tampering:

It is important to advise patients not to tamper with the packaging and to report any indications of tampering to medical professionals.

- Clinical Implications: Preserving the integrity of the packaging guarantees that the medication has not been tampered with before usage and helps prevent contamination.

How to Get Rid of Unused Medicine:

It is important to inform patients on how to properly dispose of any leftover or expired Itravil.

- Clinical Implications: Safe disposal reduces environmental effect and helps avoid accidental ingestion, particularly in homes with children.

Keeping an eye out for stability

Pharmacists and healthcare professionals should keep an eye on Itravil's stability, looking for any changes in the drug's look, smell, or integrity of packaging.

- Clinical Implications: To guarantee the safety and efficacy of the medication, any variations from the anticipated appearance or packing should be looked into.

ASPECTS TO TAKE INTO ACCOUNT FOR MEDICAL FACILITIES:

Storage Environments in Pharmacies:

The proper storage conditions for Itravil, which include controlling temperature, shielding from light, and avoiding moisture, should be followed by pharmacies.

- Clinical Implications: The quality of items provided is enhanced when pharmacy settings ensure that medication is stored under specified conditions.

Management of Inventory:

Effective inventory management systems should be put in place by healthcare facilities to keep an eye on Itravil stock levels, expiration dates, and storage conditions.

- **Clinical Implications:** Ensuring the availability of fresh stock and preventing the administration of compromised or expired pharmaceuticals are two benefits of proper inventory management.

In conclusion, it is critical for patients, pharmacists, and healthcare professionals to comprehend how Itravil is delivered, kept, and handled. For the drug to remain stable, effective, and safe, handling instructions and recommended storage conditions must be followed. Giving patients the right information about how to store and dispose of Itravil safely will enable them to actively participate in their therapy, which will improve their weight management results.

PATIENT COUNSELING INFORMATION

A key component of healthcare is patient counseling, which equips patients with the information and skills needed to utilize medications safely and effectively. Extensive patient counseling is necessary when it comes to Itravil, a medicine intended for weight control. This thorough examination will address a number of topics related to Itravil patient counseling, such as prescription details, appropriate use, possible side effects, lifestyle concerns, and the significance of continuous patient-provider communication.

Reason for Medication:

Itravil is recommended to reduce appetite and increase energy expenditure in order to help with weight management.

- Counseling Point: By knowing Itravil's main objective, patients are better able to assess the drug's significance in relation to their overall weight-management plan.

All-encompassing Method:

Itravil is usually prescribed as a component of a complete weight-management program that also includes behavioral, nutritional, and increased physical activity adjustments.

- Counseling Point: Stressing the value of a wholistic approach motivates patients to actively engage in lifestyle modifications in order to optimize Itravil's efficacy.

Nature of Prescription:

Itravil can only be purchased with a prescription, and using it should always be under a doctor's supervision.

- Counseling Point: Patients should be aware that Itravil is not a drug that can be purchased over-the-counter, which emphasizes the necessity of seeking medical advice and routine monitoring.

USAGE OF MEDICATION PROPERLY:

Instructions for Dosage:

Patients should adhere to the dosage recommendations made by their medical professional.

- Counseling Point: Stressing the value of following recommended dosages guarantees the best possible therapeutic outcomes and lowers the possibility of negative side effects.

When the Administration Will Act:

Itravil is frequently administered in order to enhance its ability to decrease hunger.

- Counseling Point: Teaching patients when to take their medications improves their ability to reduce their consumption of food.

Regular Management:

To keep their blood levels steady, patients should try to take Itravil at the same time every day.

- Counseling Point: Patients should be encouraged to create a routine since it enhances the overall effectiveness of Itravil when used consistently.

Missed Dosage Instruction:

Patients should adhere to their healthcare provider's instructions if a dose is missed. Doubling the following dosage is usually not recommended.

- Counseling Point: Potential problems with medication management can be avoided by knowing how to handle missed doses.

POSSIBLE ADVERSE REACTIONS:

Typical Adverse Reactions:

Common adverse effects that patients should be aware of include elevated heart rate, dry mouth, sleeplessness, and upset stomach.

- Counseling Point: Teaching patients about typical side effects helps them anticipate possible reactions and encourages prompt reporting to medical professionals.

Extreme Negative Reactions:

Patients should be advised to get medical help right away if they suffer from serious side effects, such as headaches, chest pain, or noticeable mood swings.

- Counseling Point: Early detection and mitigation of serious adverse responses are essential for decreasing risks.

Gradual Effects Onset:

Itravil's appetite-suppressing effects might not become fully apparent right once.

- Counseling Point: Patients should be told not to expect results right away and that weight loss may happen gradually.

Dependency and Tolerance:

Patients need to be informed that continued usage may lead to tolerance and dependency.

- Counseling Point: Early detection of tolerance enables suitable modifications to the treatment strategy. This is made possible by routine monitoring and conversation with healthcare specialists.

A LOOK AT LIFESTYLE:

Dietary Adjustments:

The best results from Itravil come from combining it with a diet high in nutrient-dense, low-calorie foods.
- Counseling Point: Patients are more likely to lose weight over time if they are encouraged to adopt a healthy, balanced diet.

Enhanced Exercise:

Engaging in regular physical activity enhances the overall effectiveness of Itravil weight management.
- Counseling Point: In accordance with their degree of fitness and the advice of their healthcare professional, patients should be encouraged to add more physical exercise to their routine.

The Significance of Hydration:

It's important to drink enough water, especially since Itravil may induce dry mouth.
- Counseling Point: Stressing the value of maintaining hydration reduces the possibility

of negative effects and promotes general wellbeing.

Use of Alcohol and Other Substances:

Patients should be counseled to refrain from using recreational drugs and to limit their alcohol intake as these may interact with Itravil.

- Counseling Point: Being aware of possible interactions helps ensure the safety of medications and encourages responsible substance use.

MONITORING SPECIFICS:

Frequent Follow-Up Meetings:

It is imperative to arrange follow-up sessions with healthcare providers in order to track advancement, modify the treatment plan, and resolve any issues.

- Counseling Point: Stressing the value of routine follow-up visits encourages continued correspondence and individualized treatment.

Vital Sign Observation:

A regular check of vital signs, such as blood pressure and heart rate, is part of the continuous evaluation of Itravil's safety.

- Counseling Point: It is important for patients to know the importance of vital sign monitoring and how it helps to ensure their health while undergoing therapy.

Progress in Losing Weight:

One of the most important components of Itravil treatment is tracking weight loss progress.

- Counseling Point: Encouraging patients to keep a record of their weight loss progress gives them a sense of achievement and assists medical professionals in making well-informed decisions regarding treatment modifications.

Psychological Surveillance:

Regular psychiatric monitoring is recommended for patients with a history of mental problems in order to identify any changes in mood or worsening of symptoms.

- Counseling Point: Prompt identification of psychological impacts enables prompt intervention and, if necessary, coordination with mental health providers.

Levels of blood glucose:

Blood glucose levels should be regularly monitored in people with diabetes mellitus.

- Counseling Point: Keeping an eye on blood sugar levels enables medical professionals to make well-informed choices on possible modifications to anti-diabetic drugs.

PARTICULAR POPULATIONS:

Getting pregnant and nursing:

Due to insufficient safety information during pregnancy and the possibility of the medication leaking into breast milk, it is not recommended for use by women who are pregnant or nursing.

- Counseling Point: It is crucial to provide patients with information about safe contraception and to prevent nursing while receiving Itravil therapy.

Children's Population:

Itravil's safety and effectiveness in pediatric populations are unknown, and using it in those less than 18 is typically not advised.

- Counseling Point: For pediatric patients, nonpharmacological therapies should be explored, and the advantages and disadvantages of any course of action should be thoroughly assessed.

Considering the Elderly:

Itravil's effects on the cardiovascular and central nervous systems may be more pronounced in elderly persons.

- Counseling Point: To reduce potential dangers, the elderly group has to get extra attention to monitoring and customized dose modifications.

CONSIDERATIONS FOR DISCONTINUATION:

Tapering Off Gradually:

Itravil should only be stopped under a doctor's supervision, and a progressive dosage reduction may be taken into consideration.

- Counseling Point: In order to reduce the possibility of experiencing withdrawal symptoms, patients should be aware of the significance of working together with their healthcare professional to make decisions about stopping treatment.

Symptoms of Withdrawal:

Itravil withdrawal symptoms, including as lethargy, depression, and appetite changes, might occur with an abrupt stop.

- Counseling Point: Patients should be informed about the possibility of experiencing withdrawal symptoms as well as the significance of promptly reporting any negative effects to their healthcare professional.

Patient counseling for Itravil is a complex process that includes information about the medication, how to take it correctly, possible side effects, lifestyle factors, monitoring measures, and considerations for stopping the drug. Fostering a cooperative and knowledgeable approach to weight management requires effective communication between patients and healthcare providers. In the ever-changing field of weight management, patient empowerment via education promotes positive outcomes and general well-being while also assisting in the safe and effective administration of Itravil.

CONCLUSION

Itravil is a pharmacological ally in the field of weight control, where lifestyle, medication, and medical advice interact in a complex way. This thorough investigation has covered every aspect of Itravil, from its pharmacological characteristics to patient counseling, exploring the complexities of its uses, mechanisms, possible side effects, and the cooperative efforts necessary for its safe and efficient use. As we come to the end of this discussion, it is necessary to summarize the most important lessons and takeaways from every aspect of Itravil's story.

Itravil's pharmacological profile highlights its function as an appetite suppressant and weight control medication, as it is marked by sympathomimetic qualities and stimulation of the central nervous system. Healthcare professionals can better manage the complexity of this medication with a foundational grasp of its pharmacodynamics, pharmacokinetics, and mechanism of action. A more knowledgeable and individualized therapy approach is facilitated by an understanding of the heterogeneity in response among individuals, the possibility of tolerance and dependency, and the requirement for a holistic approach.

Itravil is used in clinical settings for purposes other than aiding in weight loss. When included in a comprehensive weight-management approach, its potential to impact obesity-related comorbid disorders like dyslipidemia and hypertension lends further therapeutic value. The acknowledgement of Itravil as a driving force behind long-term weight control in conjunction with lifestyle adjustments highlights the significance of patient involvement and compliance with multimodal therapies.

The terrain of Itravil requires careful attention to any negative reactions and the application of proactive monitoring techniques. A proactive approach to adverse responses reduces the impact on patients and ensures early intervention for everything from gastrointestinal problems to psychiatric concerns, from cardiovascular consequences to central nervous system stimulation. Frequent monitoring which includes weight reduction progress, mental health metrics, and vital signs is the cornerstone of an adaptable and dynamic healthcare plan.

Itravil's path is anchored by patient education and counseling. There is much more to the conversation between patients and healthcare professionals than just giving out prescription drugs. It is a continuous story that encourages people to take an active role in their own health. Patient counseling is a cooperative effort that develops a sense of agency and responsibility rather than merely providing instructions on how to take medications, possible side effects, lifestyle considerations, and monitoring parameters.

Itravil's journey doesn't end with how it is administered; it also includes how it is handled, stored, and eventually stopped. The commitment to preserving the stability of the medication is highlighted by the careful attention to storage conditions, protection from environmental influences, and the emphasis on correct handling. Just as important is the thought of stopping Itravil therapy, where careful tapering, knowledge of withdrawal symptoms, and joint decision-making become essential components.

Particular populations, such as those who are pregnant or nursing, patients in pediatrics, and the elderly population, require a more delicate approach to the integration of Itravil. The dedication to patient safety and well-being is demonstrated by the recognition of contraindications, the search for alternatives, and the customization of treatment programs to account for unique vulnerabilities.

This thorough investigation of Itravil has led to a conclusion that, when applied to clinical settings, integrates patient-centered care with evidence-based methods. It is realizing that Itravil is a dynamic element in the complex fabric of customized therapy rather than just a pharmacological agent. Throughout the course of the clinical journey with Itravil, patients and healthcare professionals engage in a continuous discussion that goes beyond simply writing prescriptions to include motivation, education, and joint decision-making.

Because of the intricate pharmacology of Itravil, the possibility of side effects, and the varied ways in which it is used, healthcare professionals must adopt the roles of health educators, mentors, and collaborators. It calls for a dedication to alertness, ongoing observation, and flexibility in the face of personal variability. Itravil integration into patient care is a dynamic process that changes as patients' needs, lifestyles, and health trajectories do. It is not a static procedure.

As the story of Itravil develops, it begs for thought about possible improvements and future paths for its clinical use. Prospective research directions include examining the long-term consequences, the influence on particular subpopulations, and the identification of prediction indicators for treatment response. Technological innovations like telemedicine and digital health technologies could improve the continuity of care for those on Itravil even further.

Interdisciplinary cooperation is required to take into account a more thorough integration of Itravil into an all-encompassing obesity management paradigm. Incorporating the expertise of exercise physiologists, psychologists, and nutritionists alongside medical professionals can result in a collaborative strategy that tackles the complex aspects of obesity.

There are ethical issues to consider when traveling with Itravil. Body image, social norms, and the risk of stigma are all factors that are taken into account while prescribing and monitoring weight-management drugs. The moral responsibility is to create a caring, accepting atmosphere where people feel encouraged to pursue their health goals.

The Itravil narrative is essentially evidence of the movement in healthcare toward a patient-centered paradigm. It is a story that acknowledges the patient's autonomy, values, and goals while putting them at the center. In the framework of Itravil, the fusion of medical knowledge with patient empowerment is not only a theoretical concept but a lived reality.

The Itravil voyage is a dynamic expedition that is led by the ideals of patient education, individualized medicine, and collaborative care rather than a linear trajectory. It is a recognition that the clinical narrative embraces the complexity of human health and goes beyond the boundaries of a prescription. Empowerment, resilience, and a shared commitment to holistic well-being are the prominent themes as patients and healthcare professionals set out on this journey together.